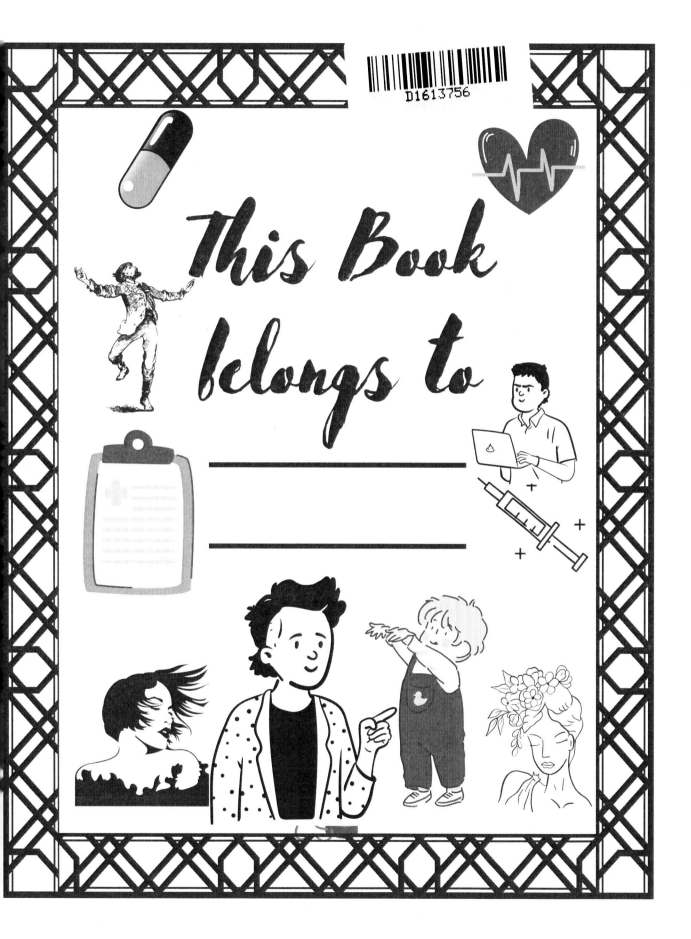

This Book belongs to

_____

_____

MY HEALTH RECORD

Name	
Date Of Birth	
Medical/Health	
Number	

Contact Name	
Address	
Phone Number 1	
Phone Number 2	

Immunizations

Date	Name

Medical Conditions

Name	Description

Medications

Name	What it is for	Dosage

Family Medical History

Medical Condition	Family Member	Family Member	Family Member	Family Member
Allergies				
Arthritis				
Auto Immune Disease				
Birth Defects				
Blood Disorder				
Cancer				
Diabetes				
Endometriosis				
Gastrointestinal Disorder				
Heart Disease				
High Blood Pressure				
High Cholesterol				
Infertility				
Kidney Disease				
Liver Disease				
Lung Disease				
Mental Illness				
Migraines				
Nerve Disorders				
Stroke / TIA				
OTHER				

Family Medical History Notes

Family Medical History

Medical Condition	Family Member	Family Member	Family Member	Family Member
Allergies				
Arthritis				
Auto Immune Disease				
Birth Defects				
Blood Disorder				
Cancer				
Diabetes				
Endometriosis				
Gastrointestinal Disorder				
Heart Disease				
High Blood Pressure				
High Cholesterol				
Infertility				
Kidney Disease				
Liver Disease				
Lung Disease				
Mental Illness				
Migraines				
Nerve Disorders				
Stroke / TIA				
OTHER				

Family Medical History Notes

Medications

Name	What it is for	Dosage

Blood Pressure and Blood Sugar Tracker

Day	Date	Time	Blood Pressure	Time	Blood Sugar	Notes
Mon						
Tue						
Wed						
Thur						
Fri						
Sat						
Sun						

Medication Tracker

Med	Dose	Date	Morning	Afternoon	Evening	Notes

Blood Pressure and Blood Sugar Tracker

Day	Date	Time	Blood Pressure	Time	Blood Sugar	Notes
Mon						
Tue						
Wed						
Thur						
Fri						
Sat						
Sun						

Medication Tracker

Med	Dose	Date	Morning	Afternoon	Evening	Notes

Blood Pressure and Blood Sugar Tracker

Day	Date	Time	Blood Pressure	Time	Blood Sugar	Notes
Mon						
Tue						
Wed						
Thur						
Fri						
Sat						
Sun						

Medication Tracker

Med	Dose	Date	Morning	Afternoon	Evening	Notes

Blood Pressure and Blood Sugar Tracker

Day	Date	Time	Blood Pressure	Time	Blood Sugar	Notes
Mon						
Tue						
Wed						
Thur						
Fri						
Sat						
Sun						

Medication Tracker

Med	Dose	Date	Morning	Afternoon	Evening	Notes

Blood Pressure and Blood Sugar Tracker

Day	Date	Time	Blood Pressure	Time	Blood Sugar	Notes
Mon						
Tue						
Wed						
Thur						
Fri						
Sat						
Sun						

Medication Tracker

Med	Dose	Date	Morning	Afternoon	Evening	Notes

Blood Pressure and Blood Sugar Tracker

Day	Date	Time	Blood Pressure	Time	Blood Sugar	Notes
Mon						
Tue						
Wed						
Thur						
Fri						
Sat						
Sun						

Medication Tracker

Med	Dose	Date	Morning	Afternoon	Evening	Notes

Blood Pressure and Blood Sugar Tracker

Day	Date	Time	Blood Pressure	Time	Blood Sugar	Notes
Mon						
Tue						
Wed						
Thur						
Fri						
Sat						
Sun						

Medication Tracker

Med	Dose	Date	Morning	Afternoon	Evening	Notes

Blood Pressure and Blood Sugar Tracker

Day	Date	Time	Blood Pressure	Time	Blood Sugar	Notes
Mon						
Tue						
Wed						
Thur						
Fri						
Sat						
Sun						

Medication Tracker

Med	Dose	Date	Morning	Afternoon	Evening	Notes

Blood Pressure and Blood Sugar Tracker

Day	Date	Time	Blood Pressure	Time	Blood Sugar	Notes
Mon						
Tue						
Wed						
Thur						
Fri						
Sat						
Sun						

Medication Tracker

Med	Dose	Date	Morning	Afternoon	Evening	Notes

Blood Pressure and Blood Sugar Tracker

Day	Date	Time	Blood Pressure	Time	Blood Sugar	Notes
Mon						
Tue						
Wed						
Thur						
Fri						
Sat						
Sun						

Medication Tracker

Med	Dose	Date	Morning	Afternoon	Evening	Notes

Blood Pressure and Blood Sugar Tracker

Day	Date	Time	Blood Pressure	Time	Blood Sugar	Notes
Mon						
Tue						
Wed						
Thur						
Fri						
Sat						
Sun						

Medication Tracker

Med	Dose	Date	Morning	Afternoon	Evening	Notes

Blood Pressure and Blood Sugar Tracker

Day	Date	Time	Blood Pressure	Time	Blood Sugar	Notes
Mon						
Tue						
Wed						
Thur						
Fri						
Sat						
Sun						

Medication Tracker

Med	Dose	Date	Morning	Afternoon	Evening	Notes

Blood Pressure and Blood Sugar Tracker

Day	Date	Time	Blood Pressure	Time	Blood Sugar	Notes
Mon						
Tue						
Wed						
Thur						
Fri						
Sat						
Sun						

Medication Tracker

Med	Dose	Date	Morning	Afternoon	Evening	Notes

Blood Pressure and Blood Sugar Tracker

Day	Date	Time	Blood Pressure	Time	Blood Sugar	Notes
Mon						
Tue						
Wed						
Thur						
Fri						
Sat						
Sun						

Medication Tracker

Med	Dose	Date	Morning	Afternoon	Evening	Notes

Blood Pressure and Blood Sugar Tracker

Day	Date	Time	Blood Pressure	Time	Blood Sugar	Notes
Mon						
Tue						
Wed						
Thur						
Fri						
Sat						
Sun						

Medication Tracker

Med	Dose	Date	Morning	Afternoon	Evening	Notes

Blood Pressure and Blood Sugar Tracker

Day	Date	Time	Blood Pressure	Time	Blood Sugar	Notes
Mon						
Tue						
Wed						
Thur						
Fri						
Sat						
Sun						

Medication Tracker

Med	Dose	Date	Morning	Afternoon	Evening	Notes

Blood Pressure and Blood Sugar Tracker

Day	Date	Time	Blood Pressure	Time	Blood Sugar	Notes
Mon						
Tue						
Wed						
Thur						
Fri						
Sat						
Sun						

Medication Tracker

Med	Dose	Date	Morning	Afternoon	Evening	Notes

Blood Pressure and Blood Sugar Tracker

Day	Date	Time	Blood Pressure	Time	Blood Sugar	Notes
Mon						
Tue						
Wed						
Thur						
Fri						
Sat						
Sun						

Medication Tracker

Med	Dose	Date	Morning	Afternoon	Evening	Notes

Blood Pressure and Blood Sugar Tracker

Day	Date	Time	Blood Pressure	Time	Blood Sugar	Notes
Mon						
Tue						
Wed						
Thur						
Fri						
Sat						
Sun						

Medication Tracker

Med	Dose	Date	Morning	Afternoon	Evening	Notes

Blood Pressure and Blood Sugar Tracker

Day	Date	Time	Blood Pressure	Time	Blood Sugar	Notes
Mon						
Tue						
Wed						
Thur						
Fri						
Sat						
Sun						

Medication Tracker

Med	Dose	Date	Morning	Afternoon	Evening	Notes

Blood Pressure and Blood Sugar Tracker

Day	Date	Time	Blood Pressure	Time	Blood Sugar	Notes
Mon						
Tue						
Wed						
Thur						
Fri						
Sat						
Sun						

Medication Tracker

Med	Dose	Date	Morning	Afternoon	Evening	Notes

Blood Pressure and Blood Sugar Tracker

Day	Date	Time	Blood Pressure	Time	Blood Sugar	Notes
Mon						
Tue						
Wed						
Thur						
Fri						
Sat						
Sun						

Medication Tracker

Med	Dose	Date	Morning	Afternoon	Evening	Notes

Blood Pressure and Blood Sugar Tracker

Day	Date	Time	Blood Pressure	Time	Blood Sugar	Notes
Mon						
Tue						
Wed						
Thur						
Fri						
Sat						
Sun						

Medication Tracker

Med	Dose	Date	Morning	Afternoon	Evening	Notes

Blood Pressure and Blood Sugar Tracker

Day	Date	Time	Blood Pressure	Time	Blood Sugar	Notes
Mon						
Tue						
Wed						
Thur						
Fri						
Sat						
Sun						

Medication Tracker

Med	Dose	Date	Morning	Afternoon	Evening	Notes

Blood Pressure and Blood Sugar Tracker

Day	Date	Time	Blood Pressure	Time	Blood Sugar	Notes
Mon						
Tue						
Wed						
Thur						
Fri						
Sat						
Sun						

Medication Tracker

Med	Dose	Date	Morning	Afternoon	Evening	Notes

Blood Pressure and Blood Sugar Tracker

Day	Date	Time	Blood Pressure	Time	Blood Sugar	Notes
Mon						
Tue						
Wed						
Thur						
Fri						
Sat						
Sun						

Medication Tracker

Med	Dose	Date	Morning	Afternoon	Evening	Notes

Blood Pressure and Blood Sugar Tracker

Day	Date	Time	Blood Pressure	Time	Blood Sugar	Notes
Mon						
Tue						
Wed						
Thur						
Fri						
Sat						
Sun						

Medication Tracker

Med	Dose	Date	Morning	Afternoon	Evening	Notes

Blood Pressure and Blood Sugar Tracker

Day	Date	Time	Blood Pressure	Time	Blood Sugar	Notes
Mon						
Tue						
Wed						
Thur						
Fri						
Sat						
Sun						

Medication Tracker

Med	Dose	Date	Morning	Afternoon	Evening	Notes

Blood Pressure and Blood Sugar Tracker

Day	Date	Time	Blood Pressure	Time	Blood Sugar	Notes
Mon						
Tue						
Wed						
Thur						
Fri						
Sat						
Sun						

Medication Tracker

Med	Dose	Date	Morning	Afternoon	Evening	Notes

Blood Pressure and Blood Sugar Tracker

Day	Date	Time	Blood Pressure	Time	Blood Sugar	Notes
Mon						
Tue						
Wed						
Thur						
Fri						
Sat						
Sun						

Medication Tracker

Med	Dose	Date	Morning	Afternoon	Evening	Notes

Blood Pressure and Blood Sugar Tracker

Day	Date	Time	Blood Pressure	Time	Blood Sugar	Notes
Mon						
Tue						
Wed						
Thur						
Fri						
Sat						
Sun						

Medication Tracker

Med	Dose	Date	Morning	Afternoon	Evening	Notes

Blood Pressure and Blood Sugar Tracker

Day	Date	Time	Blood Pressure	Time	Blood Sugar	Notes
Mon						
Tue						
Wed						
Thur						
Fri						
Sat						
Sun						

Medication Tracker

Med	Dose	Date	Morning	Afternoon	Evening	Notes

Blood Pressure and Blood Sugar Tracker

Day	Date	Time	Blood Pressure	Time	Blood Sugar	Notes
Mon						
Tue						
Wed						
Thur						
Fri						
Sat						
Sun						

Medication Tracker

Med	Dose	Date	Morning	Afternoon	Evening	Notes

Blood Pressure and Blood Sugar Tracker

Day	Date	Time	Blood Pressure	Time	Blood Sugar	Notes
Mon						
Tue						
Wed						
Thur						
Fri						
Sat						
Sun						

Medication Tracker

Med	Dose	Date	Morning	Afternoon	Evening	Notes

Blood Pressure and Blood Sugar Tracker

Day	Date	Time	Blood Pressure	Time	Blood Sugar	Notes
Mon						
Tue						
Wed						
Thur						
Fri						
Sat						
Sun						

Medication Tracker

Med	Dose	Date	Morning	Afternoon	Evening	Notes

Blood Pressure and Blood Sugar Tracker

Day	Date	Time	Blood Pressure	Time	Blood Sugar	Notes
Mon						
Tue						
Wed						
Thur						
Fri						
Sat						
Sun						

Medication Tracker

Med	Dose	Date	Morning	Afternoon	Evening	Notes

Blood Pressure and Blood Sugar Tracker

Day	Date	Time	Blood Pressure	Time	Blood Sugar	Notes
Mon						
Tue						
Wed						
Thur						
Fri						
Sat						
Sun						

Medication Tracker

Med	Dose	Date	Morning	Afternoon	Evening	Notes

Blood Pressure and Blood Sugar Tracker

Day	Date	Time	Blood Pressure	Time	Blood Sugar	Notes
Mon						
Tue						
Wed						
Thur						
Fri						
Sat						
Sun						

Medication Tracker

Med	Dose	Date	Morning	Afternoon	Evening	Notes

Blood Pressure and Blood Sugar Tracker

Day	Date	Time	Blood Pressure	Time	Blood Sugar	Notes
Mon						
Tue						
Wed						
Thur						
Fri						
Sat						
Sun						

Medication Tracker

Med	Dose	Date	Morning	Afternoon	Evening	Notes

Blood Pressure and Blood Sugar Tracker

Day	Date	Time	Blood Pressure	Time	Blood Sugar	Notes
Mon						
Tue						
Wed						
Thur						
Fri						
Sat						
Sun						

Medication Tracker

Med	Dose	Date	Morning	Afternoon	Evening	Notes

Blood Pressure and Blood Sugar Tracker

Day	Date	Time	Blood Pressure	Time	Blood Sugar	Notes
Mon						
Tue						
Wed						
Thur						
Fri						
Sat						
Sun						

Medication Tracker

Med	Dose	Date	Morning	Afternoon	Evening	Notes

Blood Pressure and Blood Sugar Tracker

Day	Date	Time	Blood Pressure	Time	Blood Sugar	Notes
Mon						
Tue						
Wed						
Thur						
Fri						
Sat						
Sun						

Medication Tracker

Med	Dose	Date	Morning	Afternoon	Evening	Notes

Blood Pressure and Blood Sugar Tracker

Day	Date	Time	Blood Pressure	Time	Blood Sugar	Notes
Mon						
Tue						
Wed						
Thur						
Fri						
Sat						
Sun						

Medication Tracker

Med	Dose	Date	Morning	Afternoon	Evening	Notes

Blood Pressure and Blood Sugar Tracker

Day	Date	Time	Blood Pressure	Time	Blood Sugar	Notes
Mon						
Tue						
Wed						
Thur						
Fri						
Sat						
Sun						

Medication Tracker

Med	Dose	Date	Morning	Afternoon	Evening	Notes

Blood Pressure and Blood Sugar Tracker

Day	Date	Time	Blood Pressure	Time	Blood Sugar	Notes
Mon						
Tue						
Wed						
Thur						
Fri						
Sat						
Sun						

Medication Tracker

Med	Dose	Date	Morning	Afternoon	Evening	Notes

Blood Pressure and Blood Sugar Tracker

Day	Date	Time	Blood Pressure	Time	Blood Sugar	Notes
Mon						
Tue						
Wed						
Thur						
Fri						
Sat						
Sun						

Medication Tracker

Med	Dose	Date	Morning	Afternoon	Evening	Notes

Blood Pressure and Blood Sugar Tracker

Day	Date	Time	Blood Pressure	Time	Blood Sugar	Notes
Mon						
Tue						
Wed						
Thur						
Fri						
Sat						
Sun						

Medication Tracker

Med	Dose	Date	Morning	Afternoon	Evening	Notes

Blood Pressure and Blood Sugar Tracker

Day	Date	Time	Blood Pressure	Time	Blood Sugar	Notes
Mon						
Tue						
Wed						
Thur						
Fri						
Sat						
Sun						

Medication Tracker

Med	Dose	Date	Morning	Afternoon	Evening	Notes

Blood Pressure and Blood Sugar Tracker

Day	Date	Time	Blood Pressure	Time	Blood Sugar	Notes
Mon						
Tue						
Wed						
Thur						
Fri						
Sat						
Sun						

Medication Tracker

Med	Dose	Date	Morning	Afternoon	Evening	Notes

Blood Pressure and Blood Sugar Tracker

Day	Date	Time	Blood Pressure	Time	Blood Sugar	Notes
Mon						
Tue						
Wed						
Thur						
Fri						
Sat						
Sun						

Medication Tracker

Med	Dose	Date	Morning	Afternoon	Evening	Notes

Blood Pressure and Blood Sugar Tracker

Day	Date	Time	Blood Pressure	Time	Blood Sugar	Notes
Mon						
Tue						
Wed						
Thur						
Fri						
Sat						
Sun						

Medication Tracker

Med	Dose	Date	Morning	Afternoon	Evening	Notes

Blood Pressure and Blood Sugar Tracker

Day	Date	Time	Blood Pressure	Time	Blood Sugar	Notes
Mon						
Tue						
Wed						
Thur						
Fri						
Sat						
Sun						

Medication Tracker

Med	Dose	Date	Morning	Afternoon	Evening	Notes

Blood Pressure and Blood Sugar Tracker

Day	Date	Time	Blood Pressure	Time	Blood Sugar	Notes
Mon						
Tue						
Wed						
Thur						
Fri						
Sat						
Sun						

Medication Tracker

Med	Dose	Date	Morning	Afternoon	Evening	Notes

Blood Pressure and Blood Sugar Tracker

Day	Date	Time	Blood Pressure	Time	Blood Sugar	Notes
Mon						
Tue						
Wed						
Thur						
Fri						
Sat						
Sun						

Medication Tracker

Med	Dose	Date	Morning	Afternoon	Evening	Notes

Blood Pressure and Blood Sugar Tracker

Day	Date	Time	Blood Pressure	Time	Blood Sugar	Notes
Mon						
Tue						
Wed						
Thur						
Fri						
Sat						
Sun						

Medication Tracker

Med	Dose	Date	Morning	Afternoon	Evening	Notes

Blood Pressure and Blood Sugar Tracker

Day	Date	Time	Blood Pressure	Time	Blood Sugar	Notes
Mon						
Tue						
Wed						
Thur						
Fri						
Sat						
Sun						

Medication Tracker

Med	Dose	Date	Morning	Afternoon	Evening	Notes

Blood Pressure and Blood Sugar Tracker

Day	Date	Time	Blood Pressure	Time	Blood Sugar	Notes
Mon						
Tue						
Wed						
Thur						
Fri						
Sat						
Sun						

Medication Tracker

Med	Dose	Date	Morning	Afternoon	Evening	Notes

Month: Year:

Medical Visits						
Date	Symptoms	Diagnosis	Tests ?	Results	Doctor's Advice	Medication

Notes:

Month: Year:

			Medical Visits			
Date	Symptoms	Diagnosis	Tests ?	Results	Doctor's Advice	Medication

Notes:

Month: Year:

			Medical Visits			
Date	Symptoms	Diagnosis	Tests ?	Results	Doctor's Advice	Medication

Notes:

Month: Year:

Medical Visits						
Date	Symptoms	Diagnosis	Tests ?	Results	Doctor's Advice	Medication

Notes:

Month: Year:

Medical Visits						
Date	Symptoms	Diagnosis	Tests ?	Results	Doctor's Advice	Medication

Notes:

Month: Year:

Medical Visits						
Date	Symptoms	Diagnosis	Tests ?	Results	Doctor's Advice	Medication

Notes:

Month: Year:

Medical Visits						
Date	Symptoms	Diagnosis	Tests ?	Results	Doctor's Advice	Medication

Notes:

Month: **Year:**

	Medical Visits					
Date	Symptoms	Diagnosis	Tests ?	Results	Doctor's Advice	Medication

Notes:

Month: Year:

Medical Visits						
Date	Symptoms	Diagnosis	Tests ?	Results	Doctor's Advice	Medication

Notes:

Month: Year:

Medical Visits						
Date	Symptoms	Diagnosis	Tests ?	Results	Doctor's Advice	Medication

Notes:

Month: Year:

Medical Visits						
Date	Symptoms	Diagnosis	Tests ?	Results	Doctor's Advice	Medication

Notes:

Month: Year:

			Medical Visits			
Date	Symptoms	Diagnosis	Tests ?	Results	Doctor's Advice	Medication

Notes:

Month: Year:

			Medical Visits			
Date	Symptoms	Diagnosis	Tests?	Results	Doctor's Advice	Medication

Notes:

Month: Year:

Medical Visits						
Date	Symptoms	Diagnosis	Tests ?	Results	Doctor's Advice	Medication

Notes:

Month: **Year:**

Medical Visits						
Date	Symptoms	Diagnosis	Tests ?	Results	Doctor's Advice	Medication

Notes:

Month: Year:

Medical Visits						
Date	Symptoms	Diagnosis	Tests ?	Results	Doctor's Advice	Medication

Notes:

Month: Year:

		Medical Visits				
Date	Symptoms	Diagnosis	Tests ?	Results	Doctor's Advice	Medication

Notes:

Month: Year:

Medical Visits						
Date	Symptoms	Diagnosis	Tests ?	Results	Doctor's Advice	Medication

Notes:

Month: Year:

Medical Visits						
Date	Symptoms	Diagnosis	Tests ?	Results	Doctor's Advice	Medication

Notes:

Month: Year:

Medical Visits						
Date	Symptoms	Diagnosis	Tests ?	Results	Doctor's Advice	Medication

Notes:

Month: **Year:**

Medical Visits						
Date	Symptoms	Diagnosis	Tests ?	Results	Doctor's Advice	Medication

Notes:

Month: Year:

Medical Visits						
Date	Symptoms	Diagnosis	Tests ?	Results	Doctor'sAdvice	Medication

Notes:

Month: Year:

Medical Visits						
Date	Symptoms	Diagnosis	Tests ?	Results	Doctor's Advice	Medication

Notes:

Month: Year:

Medical Visits						
Date	Symptoms	Diagnosis	Tests ?	Results	Doctor's Advice	Medication

Notes:

Month: Year:

Medical Visits						
Date	Symptoms	Diagnosis	Tests ?	Results	Doctor's Advice	Medication

Notes:

Month: Year:

		Medical Visits				
Date	Symptoms	Diagnosis	Tests ?	Results	Doctor's Advice	Medication

Notes:

Month: Year:

Medical Visits						
Date	Symptoms	Diagnosis	Tests ?	Results	Doctor'sAdvice	Medication

Notes:

Month: Year:

Medical Visits						
Date	Symptoms	Diagnosis	Tests ?	Results	Doctor'sAdvice	Medication

Notes:

Month: Year:

Medical Visits						
Date	Symptoms	Diagnosis	Tests ?	Results	Doctor'sAdvice	Medication

Notes:

Month: Year:

		Medical Visits				
Date	Symptoms	Diagnosis	Tests ?	Results	Doctor's Advice	Medication

Notes:

Month: Year:

Medical Visits						
Date	Symptoms	Diagnosis	Tests ?	Results	Doctor's Advice	Medication

Notes:

Month: Year:

Medical Visits						
Date	Symptoms	Diagnosis	Tests ?	Results	Doctor's Advice	Medication

Notes:

Month: Year:

			Medical Visits			
Date	Symptoms	Diagnosis	Tests ?	Results	Doctor's Advice	Medication

Notes:

Month: **Year:**

Medical Visits						
Date	Symptoms	Diagnosis	Tests ?	Results	Doctor's Advice	Medication

Notes:

Month: Year:

			Medical Visits			
Date	Symptoms	Diagnosis	Tests ?	Results	Doctor's Advice	Medication

Notes:

Month: Year:

		Medical Visits				
Date	Symptoms	Diagnosis	Tests ?	Results	Doctor's Advice	Medication

Notes:

Made in United States
North Haven, CT
26 April 2023

35904895R00057